Manual of Emergency Medical Treatment for the Dental Team

ROBERT J. BRAUN, D.D.S., M.P.H.

CHAIRMAN, DEPARTMENT OF ORAL MEDICINE
ASSOCIATE DEAN, ADVANCED EDUCATION,
RESEARCH, AND CONTINUING EDUCATION
TEMPLE UNIVERSITY SCHOOL OF DENTISTRY
PHILADELPHIA, PENNSYLVANIA

BRUCE J. CUTILLI, D.M.D., M.D.

ASSISTANT CLINICAL PROFESSOR OF ORAL AND
MAXILLOFACIAL SURGERY
TEMPLE UNIVERSITY SCHOOL OF DENTISTRY
PHILADELPHIA, PENNSYLVANIA

and

PRIVATE PRACTICE, ORAL AND MAXILLOFACIAL SURGERY
WILLOW GROVE, SPRING HOUSE, PENNSYLVANIA

Consultant

WENDY B. MCGEEHAN, B.S., R.D.H.

MANAGING DIRECTOR AND COORDINATOR
IMPLANT RESEARCH CENTER AND
ORAL MEDICINE EMERGENCY/ADMISSION CLINICS
UNIVERSITY OF PENNSYLVANIA SCHOOL OF DENTAL MEDICINE
PHILADELPHIA, PENNSYLVANIA

Manual of Emergency Medical Treatment for the Dental Team

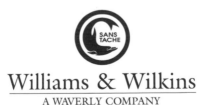

Williams & Wilkins
A WAVERLY COMPANY

BALTIMORE • PHILADELPHIA • LONDON • PARIS • BANGKOK
BUENOS AIRES • HONG KONG • MUNICH • SYDNEY • TOKYO • WROCLAW

Editor: Timothy Hisock
Managing Editor: Tanya Lazar
Marketing Manager: Adam Glazer
Project Editor: Paula C. Williams

Copyright © 1999 Williams & Wilkins

351 West Camden Street
Baltimore, Maryland 21201-2436 USA

Rose Tree Corporate Center
1400 North Providence Road
Building II, Suite 5025
Media, Pennsylvania 19063-2043 USA

Printed in the United States of America

First Edition, 1999

Library of Congress Cataloging-in-Publication Data

Braun, Robert J.
  Manual of emergency medical treatment for the dental team / Robert J. Braun, Bruce J. Cutilli.
      p.   cm.
  Includes bibliographical references.
  ISBN 0-683-30270-1
  1. Medical emergencies—Handbooks, manuals, etc.   2. Dental emergencies—Handbooks, manuals, etc.   I. Cutilli, Bruce J.   II. Title.
  [DNLM: 1. Dentistry handbooks.   2. Emergencies handbooks.   WU 49   B825m 1998]
  RC86.7.B72   1998
  616.02'5'0246176—DC21
  DNLM/DLC
  for Library of Congress   98–19198
                                                                               CIP

The publishers have made every effort to trace the copyright holders for borrowed material. If they have inadvertently overlooked any, they will be pleased to make the necessary arrangements at the first opportunity.

To purchase additional copies of this book, call our customer service department at **(800) 638-0672** or fax orders to **(800) 447-8438.** For other book services, including chapter reprints and large quantity sales, ask for the Special Sales department.

Canadian customers should call **(800) 665-1148,** or fax **(800) 665-0103.** For all other calls orig-inating outside of the United States, please call **(410) 528-4223** or fax us at **(410) 528-8550.**

Visit Williams & Wilkins on the Internet: http://www.wwilkins.com or contact our cus-tomer service department at **custserv@wwilkins.com**. Williams & Wilkins customer ser-vice representatives are available from 8:30 am to 6:00 pm, EST, Monday through Friday, for telephone access.

98 99 00 01 02
1 2 3 4 5 6 7 8 9 10

I dedicate my contribution to this book to my parents, Nancy and Vincent, whose hard work and strong value of education provided me with the foundation and inspiration to continue my studies. To my wife and best friend, Carolyn, for providing loving support and a steadying influence. To my children, Benjamin, Gregory, and Jenna, who bring immeasurable joy to our family.

BRUCE J. CUTILLI

Preface

The authors of the second edition of this manual do not intend it to be an in-depth text covering all aspects of emergency medical care. Rather, it is to be used as a companion to more comprehensive texts. We have attempted to provide a reference that will be useful at chair-side during a crisis and as an organized review of knowledge. This manual does not attempt to instruct the reader in all aspects of the mechanical skills required to treat compromised patients.

All procedures outlined are supported in the current literature. However, as in many aspects of medical care, other procedures may be appropriate and fit a particular office better. Drug dosages are calculated for the adult patient and serve only as an illustration. Specific dosages must be calculated for each treatment situation.

This text is the second iteration of a text that started out as a revision of seminar and lecture notes. Dr. Harold Gerstein was my mentor for the first edition of this text. The current text is a result of the combined efforts of the authors. Dr. Bruce Cutilli, whom I first counted only as a colleague, has become a friend during the course of this project. His knowledge and keen perceptions have added immensely to the value of this text.

Writing books can be like responding to emergencies. Things are done and at the time no one is aware of who is performing the service. However, on reflection after the event, one realizes that many people have contributed to a successful outcome. This book is the result of the hard work and encouragement of many people. Sharon Zinner believed in the project and was willing to take a chance of personal peril in working with a tardy author. Bruce Cutilli, who by keeping me on track and adding significantly to the content, ensured that this second edition would become a reality. Tanya Lazar kept the E-mail coming with suggestions to make the project flower. Scott Braun, my son, kept the process in the family and taught his dad that sons become great writers. Craig Roark, my nephew, supplied educational and artistic illustrations. Finally and especially, Karen, my wife, taught me that all things are possible.

ROBERT J. BRAUN

Contributors

Wendy B. McGeehan, B.S., R.D.H.
Managing Director and Coordinator
Implant Research Center and
    Oral Medicine Emergency/Admission Clinics
University of Pennsylvania School of Dental Medicine
Philadelphia, Pennsylvania

Scott Braun, B.S., J.D.
Former Associate of Heyl, Royster, Voelker, and Allen
Edwardsville, Illinois
Private Practice, Washington, DC

Gregory K. Spackman, D.D.S.
Associate Professor, Department of Oral and
    Maxillofacial Surgery
Dental School and Medical School
University of Texas Health Science Center
San Antonio, Texas

Craig Roark
Artist
Bethalto, Illinois

Perhaps the most valuable result of all education is the ability to make yourself do the thing you have to do, when it ought to be done, as it ought to be done, whether you like it or not.

THOMAS HUXLEY

Contents

SECTION III.
LEGAL ASPECTS TO EMERGENCY MEDICINE

SECTION IV.
TABLES

SECTION I.

Organization and Preparedness

Office Protocol

Although emergencies should not be unanticipated, they rarely occur at an opportune time. To ensure a favorable result when treating emergencies, it is necessary that all offices have a specific, rehearsed protocol for response to crisis situations. This procedure must be thoroughly explained to all office personnel, new and old. In addition, frequent review of all procedures is necessary.

It is essential that when a crisis occurs, the event is managed as efficiently as possible. Time must not be wasted, and duplication of effort should be minimized. Dental offices run efficiently because specific duties and roles are assigned to staff members for various functions. Specific assigned staff roles in an emergency situation are critical for ensuring that the patient is treated in an efficient and timely fashion.

Assignment of roles during a crisis should be based on an assessment of each staff member's abilities to function in emergency situations. Many health-care providers cannot function well in crisis situations. This statement is not meant to be pejorative; it is only meant to illustrate that a competent chair-side assistant may not be the person to assist in a medical emergency situation, whereas a receptionist may function extremely well under stressful conditions.

One person must be responsible for directing the activities of all personnel involved in treating the emergency. This person is usually the doctor. Another team member should remain to assist in treating the patient. When directed, a third team member or the first assistant should summon a physician or rescue squad.

Everyone in the office should know the location of the emergency oxygen supply and drug kit. These should always be kept in the same place. Telephone numbers of a rescue squad, nearest hospital, and a nearby physician who has agreed to respond if needed should be conspicuously posted by all telephones. All office personnel should be certified in cardiopulmonary resuscitation techniques at least to the basic rescuer level.

Physiologic crises can only be favorably resolved if thought about and planned for in advance. The "ostrich" approach to medical emergencies will not succeed. A well-trained and rehearsed staff will.

OFFICE STAFF ROLES

During a medical emergency, two general areas of concern must be addressed. These are coordinating communication with the EMS system and assisting the primary responder (usually the doctor) with the clinical management of the emergency. There are various other responsibilities that must also be assigned. These responsibilities and a suggested assignment protocol follow.

Receptionist: Prevention

A completed physical status questionnaire should be obtained for review by the doctor.

Pertinent questions about the following can prevent emergencies: allergies, previous episodes of syncope, current medications, and current medical conditions such as diabetes, hypertension, or cardiovascular disease.

Telephone numbers for the EMS system should be clearly posted on the telephone. Other telephone numbers that should be posted on or near the telephone include (1) the ambulance service if different than 911, and (2) the hospital emergency room to which patients will be transported. This is critical for information to be provided to the emergency room physicians if the EMS responders are not paramedics.

Chair-Side Assistant: Observation

The assistant should be able to recognize common symptoms of impending problems, including the following:

Change in skin color

Change in speech (pace, slurring, etc.)

Change in mobility

The assistant should also know **exactly** where all emergency equipment is located, including the following:

Oxygen

Emergency kit

Aids for physical protection of the patient

Additionally, the assistant should know how to prepare and use the emergency equipment (e.g., administration of positive pressure oxygen). He or she should also know the basics of CPR.

Hygienist or Second Responder (Additional Doctors in the Office): Responsibility

This must be a person who has had formal education in anatomy, physiology, and pathology. This person is responsible for managing the elements of the emergency that are not directly related to treating the patient, such as determining if the EMS system should be activated, keeping an exact record of the event, and sharing responsibility for case management.

Record of Emergency Care

Patient Name_____ Date _____ Time _____

Address _____

_____

Phone: Home _____ Work _____

Health-Care Providers Present:_____

Treating Doctors: _____

_____

_____

Assistants: _____

_____

_____

Past Medical History:_____

_____

_____

_____

_____

Medications:

Name	Dose

Allergies: _____

_____

_____

Circumstances: _____

_____

_____

_____

_____

_____

_____

_____

Vital Signs:

Time	BP	Pulse	Respir	Oxygen Flow (l/min)	Patient Position	Medications Given

Treatment Given:

_____

_____

_____

_____

Ambulance: Time Called _____ **Called by** _____

Arrived_____

Patient Transported to _____

Departure Time _____

Next of Kin Called _____ **Time**_____

Patient Condition When Transported: _____

_____

_____

_____

_____

Patient Belongings Given to_____

Patient Driven Home by _____ **(Relation)** _____

Follow-Up Phone Call _____ **(Time)** _____

Dentist/Physician Signature_____

Suggested Components of an Emergency Kit

EQUIPMENT

Essential

Portable oxygen, at least an E-size tank
Means of administering positive pressure ventilation
    Bag mask
    Automatic system
    Both must be equipped with a **clear** face mask
Airways
    Oropharyngeal (Fig. 1)
    Nasopharyngeal (Fig. 2)
High-volume suction
Stethoscope
Sphygmomanometer
Thermometer (disposable, nonbreakable)

Desirable

Large T&A suction tip
Pliable suction catheters
Alcohol swabs
Sterile disposable needles, assortment of gauges
Sterile disposable syringes, 5 and 10 mL
Cricothyrotomy needle or 13-gauge short straight needle
IV infusion sets
Magill or other straight forceps
Tourniquets
Tape
Penlight

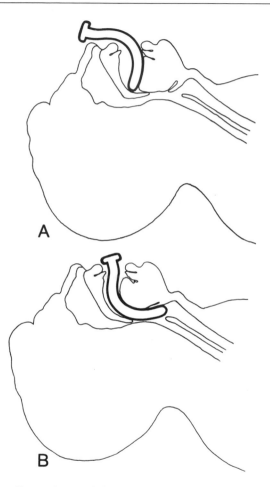

Figure 1. The oropharyngeal airway. **A.** Airway is inserted between the patient's teeth, with the convexity pointing toward the patient's feet. **B.** As the airway passes the back of the tongue, it is rotated into its resting position so the concavity points toward the patient's feet.

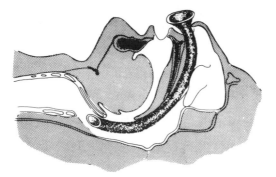

Figure 2. The nasopharyngeal airway. (Reprinted with permission from Warner A. Nasopharyngeal airway: a facilitated access to the trachea. Ann Intern Med 1971;75:594.)

DRUGS

Essential

Amyl nitrite inhalant
Aromatic ammonia inhalant
Epinephrine 1:1000, prepackaged
Glucose, sugar or cake decoration tube
Nitroglycerin
Oxygen

Desirable

Diazepam (Valium)—prepackaged syringe
Diphenhydramine (Benadryl)
Glucagon
Injectable dextrose
Proventil/Ventolin
Steroid

Advanced Cardiac Life Support

Furosemide
IV solution—Ringer's or D5W
Morphine sulfate

SUGGESTED COMPONENTS OF AN EMERGENCY KIT

Drug	Generic Name	Mode of Administration	Action
Essential			
Amyl-nitrite	Amyl-nitrite	Inhalant	Relaxes smooth muscle
Aromatic ammonia	Ammonia	Inhalant	Mechanical/chemical irritant
Epinephrine	Epinephrine	1:1000 IM or SQ 1:10,000 IV or IM	Cardiac stimulant; bronchodilator
Glucose/dextrose	Sugar/cake decoration	Oral	Elevates blood sugar
	Glucose	50 mL 50% solution IM or IV	Antihypoglycemic
Nitroglycerine	Nitroglycerin	Sublingual tablets	Relaxes smooth muscle; dilates coronary arteries
Desirable			
Benadryl	Diphenhydramine	50 mg IM or IV	Antihistamine
Glucagon	Glucagon	2–3 mg IV or IM	Antihypoglycemic
Proventil/Ventolin	Albuterol/proventil/terbutaline	Aerosol 1–2 puffs	Bronchodilator
Solu-Cortef	Steroid/hydrocortisone Sodium succinate	100 mg IM or IV	Anti-inflammatory
Valium	Diazepam	5–10 mg IM	Anticonvulsant
Advanced Cardiac Life Support			
Lasix	Furosemide	20 mg IV or IM	Diuretic
Morphine	Morphine sulfate	10–15 mg IM	Analgesic/sedative
Solution	Ringer's or D5W	IV	Adds fluid volume
Theophylline	Theophylline/aminophylline	Aerosol 1–2 puffs	Stimulates respiration, increases cardiac rate and force of contraction; diuresis; relaxes bronchial smooth muscle

History and Physical Examination

The medical history and physical examination can be the most important part of the health-care process. The information a health-care provider obtains in the medical history can be vital in preventing, diagnosing early, or easily treating a medical emergency. Other benefits of obtaining a thorough medical history and physical examination include (1) the patient perceives a greater interest in his or her total health, (2) the health-care provider realizes a greater sense of personal, professional satisfaction in his or her work, and (3) complete medical legal documentation is obtained.

Components of a comprehensive medical history and physical examination are listed in the following sections.

HISTORY

Identifying Data
Age, race, sex, and occupation.

Chief Complaint (CC)
Signs or symptoms described in the patient's own words.

History of the Present Illness (HPI)
In a narrative style and in a chronological sequence, the patient describes what has been occurring with the current medical problems.

Past Medical History (PMH)

    General health

    Childhood diseases

    Adult diseases

    Hospitalization

    Surgery

Medications

List of medications, doses, and dosing frequencies.

Allergies

List allergies or no known drug allergies (NKDA).

Social History

Alcohol use, smoking (number of packs, how many years), drug use, occupation.

Family History

Family history of similar illnesses (hypertension, diabetes, cancer).

Review of Symptoms

Included for completeness, this review can be quite extensive. However, most dental situations require a limited review.

PHYSICAL EXAMINATION

General Appearance/Assessment

Vital Signs

Blood pressure, pulse, temperature, and respiration rate.

Head and Neck

Head: Scalp, muscles of mastication, sinuses

Eyes: Pupil size, symmetry, and reactivity; extraocular movements; soft tissue color (lids and conjunctiva)

Ears: Exterior structures, discharge

Nose: Symmetry, discharge

Mouth and Oral Structures: Soft tissue color, contours, moistness

Neck: Lymph nodes, salivary glands, thyroid, carotid pulses

Thorax and Lungs

Palpation, percussion, and auscultation.

Cardiovascular

Neck veins

Heart and Pericardium: inspection and palpation

Auscultation

Peripheral pulses

Abdomen

Inspection, auscultation (bowel sounds), percussion, and palpation.

Extremities and Joints

Upper, lower, and back.

Neurologic Screening

Mental status (change in mental status)

Speech

Gait

Cranial nerves

Motor function

Sensory

Reflexes

Genital and Rectal

Deferred.

The above description of a sample history and physical examination is intended to be a guide in evaluation of a dental patient and is not intended to substitute for a comprehensive medical examination.

Procedures Used in All Emergency Situations

In dentistry and other medical specialties, patient assessment and disease diagnosis are usually the first steps taken in designing a treatment plan. Medical emergency situations require an approach that begins with treatment decisions rather than specific diagnostic approaches.

Stabilization of the patient is the first priority during physiologic crises. No matter what the cause of the event, it is essential to assess and support essential life functions. Therefore, the following steps should be taken for all patients who are experiencing an actual or potential life-threatening situation.

Position the patient in a supine position, head lower than feet if possible

Do not attempt to move the patient from the dental chair

It is possible to perform effective CPR while the patient is in the dental chair, and it is easier to access and immobilize an arm if intravenous medications are required

If the patient is conscious, he or she may be more comfortable in a sitting position

Support and reassure the patient

Provide oxygen (Fig. 3)

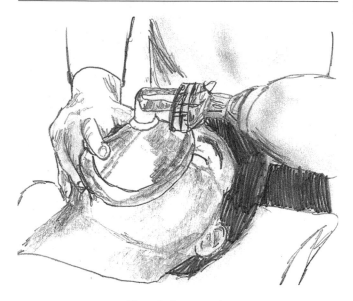

Figure 3. Oxygen mask.

Maintain an open airway

Check the patient's vital signs

Be prepared to begin CPR

Check skin color, temperature, and moisture

Evaluate information and arrive at a tentative diagnosis

Provide definitive treatment

Adult Emergency Care

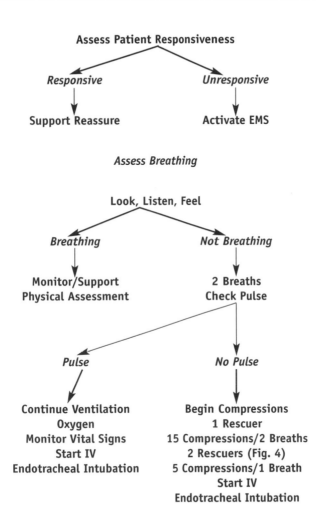

Assess Patient Responsiveness

Responsive   *Unresponsive*

Support Reassure   **Activate EMS**

Assess Breathing

Look, Listen, Feel

Breathing   *Not Breathing*

Monitor/Support   **2 Breaths**
Physical Assessment   **Check Pulse**

Pulse   *No Pulse*

Continue Ventilation   **Begin Compressions**
Oxygen   **1 Rescuer**
Monitor Vital Signs   **15 Compressions/2 Breaths**
Start IV   **2 Rescuers (Fig. 4)**
Endotracheal Intubation   **5 Compressions/1 Breath**
Start IV
Endotracheal Intubation

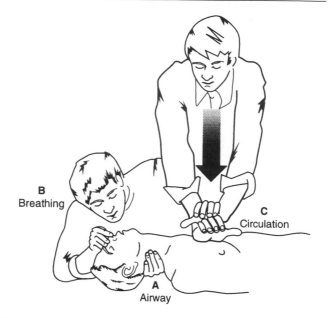

Figure 4. Two-rescuer cardiopulmonary resuscitation cycle. (Reprinted with permission from Collins VJ. Physiologic and pharmacologic bases of anesthesia. Baltimore: Williams & Wilkins, 1996. Redrawn from Paraskos JA. Guidelines for cardiopulmonary resuscitation and emergency cardiac care. JAMA 1992;268:2178.)

Infant and Child Basic Cardiac Life Support

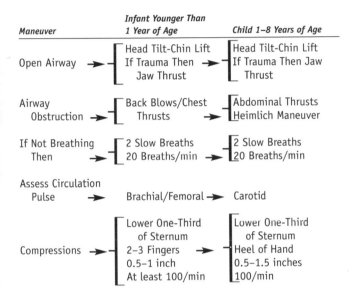

Maneuver	Infant Younger Than 1 Year of Age	Child 1–8 Years of Age
Open Airway	Head Tilt-Chin Lift If Trauma Then Jaw Thrust	Head Tilt-Chin Lift If Trauma Then Jaw Thrust
Airway Obstruction	Back Blows/Chest Thrusts	Abdominal Thrusts Heimlich Maneuver
If Not Breathing Then	2 Slow Breaths 20 Breaths/min	2 Slow Breaths 20 Breaths/min
Assess Circulation Pulse	Brachial/Femoral	Carotid
Compressions	Lower One-Third of Sternum 2–3 Fingers 0.5–1 inch At least 100/min	Lower One-Third of Sternum Heel of Hand 0.5–1.5 inches 100/min

SECTION II.

Specific Emergencies

INTRO

The adrenal gland consists of two discrete regions. The adrenal cortex primarily produces endogenous steroids. The medulla produces and secretes epinephrine and norepinephrine (catecholamines). Hypofunction of the adrenal cortex (Addison's disease) results in decreased cortisol production. Cortisol is vital in helping the body react to stressful situations. Individuals with decreased cortisol production cannot respond to stress and risk cardiovascular collapse and possible death. Patients taking exogenous steroids may have adrenal medullary suppression with decreased cortisol production and therefore an inability to produce cortisol when stress is encountered. Many health-care providers recommend increasing the level of exogenous steroids before undergoing any stressful procedure.

Adrenal Crisis

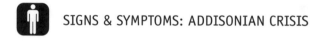 SIGNS & SYMPTOMS: ADDISONIAN CRISIS

Shocklike symptoms (cardiovascular collapse)

    Hypotension

    Bradycardia

    Fever

    Respiratory depression

Hypercalcemia

Lethargy

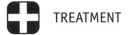 TREATMENT

Terminate treatment

Monitor and record vital signs

Place patient in Trendelenburg's position

Assess and support airway, breathing, and circulation—basic life support (BLS)

Provide supplemental oxygen

Start IV hydration with normal saline or D5NSS

Administer supplemental hydrocortisone IV or IM

Transport patient to nearest hospital emergency room

Airway Obstruction

 INTRO

It is unlikely that an unexpected airway obstruction will occur while a patient is being treated. However, unexpected airway obstructions may occur while patients or others are in the reception room or other areas of the dental office. Upper airway obstruction generally is reversible, and total obstruction is rare. The most common cause of upper airway obstruction is unconsciousness. In this situation the jaw retrudes, causing occlusion of the airway by the patient's tongue. The epiglottis can also occlude the airway.

Upper airway obstruction can cause loss of consciousness and cardiac arrest. Airway obstruction must be considered as a differential diagnosis in anyone who stops breathing.

Diagnosis of partial versus complete obstruction is critical and must be done rapidly to prevent serious complications from total anoxia. If a person is making coughing or other noises, the obstruction is partial. If no noises are made although the patient is attempting to cough or talk, the obstruction is complete.

SIGNS & SYMPTOMS

Choking

Gagging

Violent inspiratory efforts

Flushed face

Extreme anxiety

Cyanosis

Cardiovascular collapse

Airway Obstruction

 TREATMENT

Position head (Fig. 5)

Remove foreign object

    Sweeping motion of fingers

    Magil or straight forceps

    Suction

Perform abdominal thrusts/Heimlich maneuver

If the above procedures are unsuccessful after repeated attempts, cricothyrotomy is indicated.

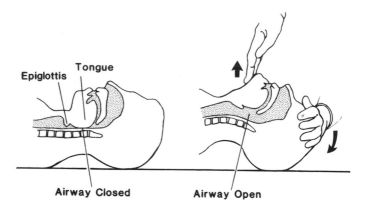

Figure 5. Chin lift to open airway. (Reprinted with permission from Wilkins EM. Clinical practice of the dental hygienist. 7th ed. Baltimore: Williams & Wilkins, 1994.)

CRICOTHYROTOMY

Rationale

Noninvasive techniques for removing objects from an airway are usually effective. However, when noninvasive techniques are not effective or when laryngeal or epiglottis swelling is present, an invasive procedure may be the only recourse in establishing a patent airway. The surgical procedure com-

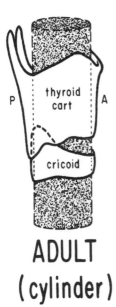

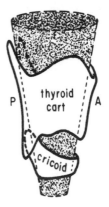

ADULT
(cylinder)

INFANT
(funnel)

Figure 6. The structures of the adult and infant larynx. (Reprinted with permission from Cote C, Todres ID. The pediatric airway. In: Ryan JF, Todres ID, Cote C, et al., eds. A practice of anesthesia for infants and children. New York: Grune and Stratton, 1988.)

monly known as cricothyrotomy is used in emergency situations. Tracheostomies are generally done when long-term airway maintenance is necessary.

The narrowest portion of the adult trachea is the larynx. Most obstructions occur in this area. A small object will usually pass through the trachea and lodge in either of the two main-stem bronchi. This is usually not acutely life-threatening. Cricothyrotomy will usually provide an opening into the trachea below an obstruction.

Anatomy

The thyroid cartilage is the largest tracheal cartilage. The cricoid is the second-largest cartilage and the only other complete ring. A membrane connects the two cartilaginous rings.

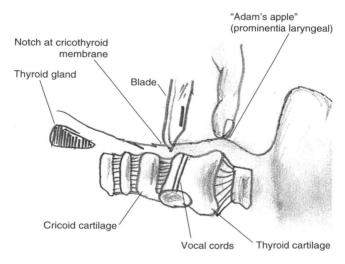

Figure 7. Cricothyrotomy.

Technique

Locate the thyroid prominence (Adam's apple) at the midline. Moving a finger inferiorly, a depression will be felt; this is the cricothyroid ligament (Figs. 6 and 7). The cricoid cartilage is located inferior to the ligament. When palpated, the cricoid cartilage feels somewhat like a half-round, plain wedding band.

The cricothyroid membrane is punctured by using a scalpel or large-bore (13-gauge) needle (Fig. 7). This causes little discomfort to the unconscious patient. Bleeding is minimal, coming from the skin incision only. It is unlikely that the esophagus will be entered as the cricoid cartilage encircles the trachea. Patency of the opening is maintained by stabilizing the needle with tape. If a scalpel is used, the handle should be inserted into the opening and rotated slightly.

If spontaneous respiration does not begin, positive pressure ventilation must be started. Any time surgical intervention is used to establish an airway, the patient must be transported to the hospital.

Anaphylaxis/Allergy

 INTRO

A hypersensitive state that results from exposure to an allergen defines allergy. Allergic reactions range in clinical manifestation from an immediate life-threatening condition seen within seconds of an exposure to delayed type reactions, the manifestations of which may not be seen until hours or days after the exposure.

Immediate or anaphylactic reactions that occur in the dental office pose the greatest risk to patients and are those that concern dentists most. Anaphylactic reactions usually result from drug administration or reaction to an allergen in impression material or other materials used in the oral cavity. The most frequent cause is related to drug administration.

Generalized anaphylaxis is the most life-threatening and dramatic allergic reaction. Death can occur in minutes if appropriate treatment is not instituted. Signs and symptoms of anaphylaxis vary; however, they generally affect the skin, smooth muscle, and respiratory and cardiovascular systems. Anaphylactic shock is the term used when consciousness is lost as a result of hypotension from an anaphylactic reaction. Symptoms usually spread beginning with the skin, followed by the eyes, nose, and gastrointestinal system and then the respiratory system; finally, cardiovascular symptoms develop.

Prompt therapy can stop the reaction. Epinephrine is the drug of choice in an immediate reaction because the onset of action is almost immediate. Administration of corticosteroids is to prevent relapse; the onset of action of steroids is 6 hours.

If epinephrine and antihistamine administration do not reverse obstruction of the airway, intubation or cricothyrotomy may be necessary.

Anaphylaxis/Allergy

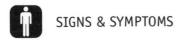 SIGNS & SYMPTOMS

Urticaria—itching, flushing, hives

Rash

Rhinitis

Bronchospasm

Laryngeal edema

Weak pulse—syncope

Loss of consciousness

Cardiac arrest

Anaphylaxis/Allergy

 TREATMENT OF AN ACUTE REACTION

Basic life support

Epinephrine, 0.3 to 0.5 mL of 1:1000 SQ IM, intralingual or sublingual—repeat if no response

Oxygen

Diphenhydramine, 50 mL IM

Corticosteroid

CPR

Airway management—intubation or cricothyrotomy

INTRO

Reaction to local anesthesia can be varied in extent and severity. However, most reactions are a result of either the local anesthetic agent itself or the vasoconstrictor within the formulation. Although today's local anesthetics have a wide therapeutic index, toxicity can occur—most commonly from rapid intravascular injection. Reactions to local anesthetics can occur as quickly as 30 to 60 seconds or as slowly as 1 hour after injection. Local anesthetic dosing should be calculated based on the patient's physical condition and body weight (see dosing guidelines table in Section IV).

Anesthesia Reactions

 SIGNS & SYMPTOMS OF LOCAL ANESTHETIC TOXICITY

Light-headedness

Changes in vision/blurred vision

Change in mental status

Confusion

Disorientation

Drowsiness

Headache

Anxiety

Tinnitus

Slurred speech

Tremors

Nausea/vomiting

Diaphoresis

Nystagmus

Seizures

Bradycardia

Tachypnea

SIGNS & SYMPTOMS OF VASOCONSTRICTOR TOXICITY

Anxiety

Tachycardia/palpitations

Restlessness

Headache

Tachypnea

Chest pain

Dysrhythmias

Cardiac arrest

Anesthesia Reactions

TREATMENT OF LOCAL ANESTHETIC TOXICITY

Initially, the dental practitioner must administer basic cardiac life support

Assess and support airway, breathing, and circulation (BCS)

Supportive treatment may be indicated

The airway should be opened

Supplemental oxygen should be given

For severe reactions, the patient should be transported to the local hospital emergency room as soon as possible

IF TRAINED IN ADVANCED CARDIAC LIFE SUPPORT

Start IV fluids

Support blood pressure with vasopressors

Treat arrhythmias

Treat allergic reaction with diphenhydramine (50 mg IV/IM) and/or epinephrine (0.3 mL 1:1000 or 3 mL 1:10,000 IV) for adults

Titrate diazepam to effect if there is persistent seizure activity

Transport the patient to the local hospital emergency room as soon as possible

INTRO

Angina pectoris is chest pain caused by temporary myocardial ischemia without damage to the heart muscle. This ischemia is due to the narrowed coronary arteries' inability to supply the myocardium with sufficient blood to meet the heart's demand for oxygen during times of stress. This narrowing can be caused by atherosclerotic vessel disease, coronary artery vasospasm, or a combination of both entities.

As with many other disease states, a detailed medical history is vital to preventing these occurrences. The astute health-care provider will attempt to quantify the extent and pattern of the disease (what types of activities have caused symptoms in the past) before beginning treatment.

Angina Pectoris

 SIGNS & SYMPTOMS

Chest pain brought on by myocardial stress (increased myocardial oxygen demand)

Left center or center chest location

Chest fullness

Burning

Tightness

Pain can radiate to neck, left arm, jaw, back, shoulder, and epigastrium

Weakness

Dyspnea

Nausea

Diaphoresis

Pain can last up to 20 minutes; however, prolonged discomfort should be evaluated in an appropriate emergency medical facility

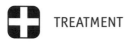 TREATMENT

Avoid situations that can produce increased myocardial oxygen demand

Stop procedure and allow the patient to rest

Monitor vital signs repeatedly

Place the patient in a semireclined position

Provide supplemental oxygen

Administer sublingual nitroglycerin (0.4 mg) every 5 minutes for three doses; if symptoms are not relieved, assume that the patient is having a myocardial infarction and transport him or her to an appropriate emergency medical facility

Asthma

 INTRO

Asthma is actually a group of illnesses producing a reversible hyperreactivity of large and small airways. Individuals may react to many types of stimuli. The incidence in the general population seems to be rising, with many young patients also suffering from other allergic conditions. Triggering factors include pollen, stress, cold, upper respiratory tract infections, exercise, animal fur, and nonsteroidal anti-inflammatory medications.

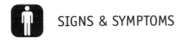 SIGNS & SYMPTOMS

Wheezing

Shortness of breath

Cough

Sputum production

Use of accessory muscles for breathing

Tachycardia

Asthma

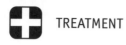 TREATMENT

The primary objective is to improve ventilation by reducing or eliminating bronchospasm

The patient should be removed from local irritants

β-adrenergic aerosolized bronchodilators should be administered

> Inhalers: Albuterol-Ventolin, Proventil two to three puffs every 4 to 6 hours; Terbutaline

The following vital signs should be monitored

> Blood pressure

> Pulse

> Blood oxygenation if available (Pulse Ox)

Supplemental oxygen should be provided

Epinephrine, 0.3 mL 1:1000 IM or SQ, should be given and repeated every 15 minutes as needed

IV theophylline should be administered

Anti-inflammatory medications such as corticosteroids or cromolyn should be given for longer-term therapy

Cardiac Dysrhythmias

 INTRO

Cardiac dysrhythmias most often present in the dental office as heart palpitations. These palpitations are often a result of anxiety about the dental procedure. Other times, however, dysrhythmias can be a result of epinephrine given in the local anesthetic or of some underlying cardiac conditions. Occasionally, simple reassurance will calm the nervous patient; however, individuals with more severe problems will require more extensive intervention to treat dysrhythmia.

Cardiac Dysrhythmias

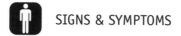 SIGNS & SYMPTOMS

Racing heart (tachycardia)

Irregular heart beat

Apprehension

Chest discomfort

Light-headedness

Chest pain (if situation worsens)

TREATMENT

Monitor vital signs continually

Place patient in a reclined position

Administer supplemental oxygen

Activate emergency medical system

Monitor ECG if available

Start IV fluids

Initiate appropriate advanced cardiac life support protocol if the patient's condition worsens (i.e., there is a drop in blood pressure or change in the level of consciousness)

Cerebrovascular Accident/Stroke

 INTRO

A cerebrovascular accident is any process that acutely interferes with blood flow to the brain. A prolonged ischemic event results in an infarction of a portion of the brain. This infarction can result in a new neurologic deficit.

The three major causes of stroke are arterial thrombosis, embolism, and hemorrhage of the vasculature. Hemorrhage of any intracranial vessel can produce a mass effect resulting in occlusion of surrounding major arteries. The internal carotid and vertebrobasilar vascular system supply the majority of the blood to the brain. A vascular occlusive incident in any of these specific vessel produces a well-defined, predictable neurologic deficit.

Cerebrovascular Accident/Stroke

 SIGNS & SYMPTOMS

Headache

Confusion

Vertigo

Nausea/vomiting

Change in mental status

Alteration in consciousness

Alteration in vision

Alteration in speech

Extremity weakness

Facial weakness

Hypertension

Cerebrovascular Accident/Stroke

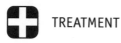 TREATMENT

Assess and monitor vital signs

Initiate basic cardiac life support as indicated

Administer supplemental oxygen if patient becomes unconscious or shows signs of respiratory difficulty

Place patient in a supine position with head slightly elevated

Transport patient to the nearest hospital for comprehensive evaluation and treatment

Congestive Heart Failure

 INTRO

Congestive heart failure is defined as the failure of the cardiac ventricles to pump blood efficiently to the body and lungs, resulting in pulmonary edema and peripheral edema. This results in overfilling of the venous system. Pulmonary edema can be a result of either lung disease or left ventricular failure. Causes of acute onset of congestive heart failure are new arrhythmias, new myocardial infarction, acute volume overload, and stress.

Congestive Heart Failure

 SIGNS & SYMPTOMS

Shortness of breath

Exertional dyspnea

Fatigue

Orthopneas (two to three pillows needed to sleep)

Cough

Rales (crackles) at lung bases

Edema—right-sided failure

Plural effusion (fluid in the lungs)

Jugular venous distention

Pink frothy sputum

S_3 and/or S_4 heart sounds

TREATMENT

Correct the underlying cause

Stress

Infection

Environmental conditions (heat)

Administer supplemental oxygen

Monitor vital signs repeatedly

Discontinue procedure

Reduce cardiac work by having the patient rest in a semireclined position

Transport the patient to an appropriate emergency facility

ADVANCED TREATMENT OF ACUTE PULMONARY EDEMA

Reduce excess fluid

Diuretics

IV furosemide (must monitor electrolytes)

Improve cardiac output

Positive inotropes

Morphine sulfate

Vasodilators

IV aminophylline

Drug-Related Emergencies

 INTRO

The use of therapeutic agents is increasing in dentistry. These agents (antibiotics, analgesics) can precipitate a physiologic crisis. Generally, these present as allergic or toxic reactions that are discussed elsewhere. Inappropriate use of drugs (drug abuse) can also lead to emergent situations. Abuse potential exists with the use of almost any drug; however, certain drugs are more commonly used and therefore more likely to present problems in the dental office.

Drugs most commonly abused are those that have actions on the central nervous system (CNS) (such as alcohol and cocaine), which alter perception. This action contributes to the allure of these agents for recreational use.

Since 1975, there has been a slow decline in recreational drug use in the United States. However, alcohol consumption and marijuana smoking are on the rise, particularly among high school students. Cocaine is the most common single cause of drug-related emergency department visits in the United States, accounting for more than twice the number of reports to the Drug Abuse Warning Network (DAWN) as heroin, the next most common drug. The National Household Survey found that in 1994, almost 22 million Americans aged 12 and older had used cocaine at least once. Approximately 3.7 million had used cocaine during the past year, and 1.3 million had used cocaine in the previous month. Whereas the increase in drug-related emergencies may be the result of increased use of drugs in combination, particularly alcohol, the primary cause appears to be cocaine.

Drug-Related Emergencies

Dentists must be aware of the signs and symptoms of drug abuse. Dentists are primary-care health providers and thus have a responsibility to patients to do no harm in providing care. Therefore, dentists must also be aware of drug interactions and of patients' abilities to follow written and verbal directions regarding postoperative medications.

Drug-Related Emergencies

 SIGNS & SYMPTOMS

CNS and cardiac dysfunction are the major signs and symptoms indicating that immediate therapy is necessary. The most common CNS indication for treatment are seizures. Cardiac dysfunction usually presents first with dysrhythmias and QRS widening.

Symptoms of Drugs Acting on the CNS

Stimulation

Headache

Nausea

Vomiting

Vertigo

Twitching of small muscles, especially facial and finger tics

Hallucinations

    Increased blood pressure

    Slow or rapid pulse rate

    Pallor

Increase in respiratory rate and depth

Elevated body temperature

    Euphoria

    Elation

    Garrulous talk

Agitation

Apprehension

Excitation

Restlessness

Emotional instability

Advanced Stimulation

Generalized seizures and status epilepticus

Decreased responsiveness to all stimuli

Incontinence

Hypertension

Tachycardia

Ventricular dysrhythmias

Weak, rapid pulse

Rapid, deep, irregular breathing

Depression (Premorbid State)

Coma

Pupils fixed and dilated

Flaccid paralysis

Circulatory failure

Cardiac arrest

Respiratory failure

Cyanosis

Lethargy

Stupor

Coma

Drug-Related Emergencies

 TREATMENT

Hypotension with evidence of shock in nonresponsive individuals is an indication for parenteral fluid therapy. Naloxone hydrochloride 0.1–0.4 mg IM/IV (Narcan) is indicated in those individuals who are experiencing a narcotic overdose reaction.

Basic life support

CPR

INTRO

Hyperglycemia is a condition of increased blood sugar. It is one of two acutely life-threatening complications of diabetes. Although relatively slow to develop, this condition, if not treated, can result in diabetic coma and death (see section on hypoglycemia, the other acutely life-threatening condition of diabetes).

Hyperglycemia

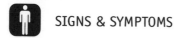 SIGNS & SYMPTOMS

Deep, labored (Kussmaul) respirations

Sweet, fruity breath

Dry, warm skin

Rapid, weak pulse

Thirst

Lassitude

Headache

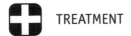 **TREATMENT**

Terminate procedure

Administer glucose

    Oral—paste or drink

    IV—D5W

Perform basic life support

Transport patient to the hospital

Hypertension

 INTRO

It is unlikely that hypertensive crises will be seen in the dental office. Most often, hypertension is an underlying cause for the development of other physiologic crises. Recognition of a hypertensive crisis does not depend as much on the absolute pressure readings as it does on clinical signs and symptoms.

Recording blood pressure during an emergency is essential; however, the value of these readings is diminished if a baseline blood pressure is not recorded as part of the pretreatment physical assessment. A blood pressure of 145/95 mm Hg may be unremarkable in a person who is being treated for severe hypertension or has no symptoms, whereas a patient experiencing symptoms or in whom a reading of this magnitude is unusual may require urgent treatment or referral.

Altered physical states due to high blood pressure can present as emergencies or urgencies. In hypertensive emergencies, the rate of rise and absolute value of the blood pressure are critical. Emergencies related to increased blood pressure result from end organ disease or the action of therapeutic or recreational drugs. These situations must be treated immediately in a hospital.

An urgency is present when an elevated blood pressure reading is obtained in the absence of any signs or symptoms. Absolute pressure readings in urgent situations may be higher than those in emergency situations. It is the presence of end organ damage or symptoms that determines the need for emergent versus referral care.

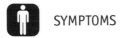 SYMPTOMS

Headache

Vomiting

Change in mental status

Visual disturbance

Seizures

Shock

Stroke

Hypertension

 SIGNS

Category	Systolic Blood Pressure (mm Hg)	Diastolic Blood Pressure (mm Hg)
Normal	<140	<90
Hypertensive		
Mild	140–159	90–104
Moderate	140–159	105–114
Severe	>159	>114

TREATMENT

Treatment of sequelae of hypertensive emergencies is described in other sections of this text. If primary blood pressure control is the objective, this must be done in a hospital by physicians. Treatment must be performed carefully to prevent a precipitous drop in pressure.

Hyperventilation

 INTRO

The result of hyperventilation is an imbalance in the ratio of blood oxygen and blood carbon dioxide levels. This condition may be produced by either rapid or excessively deep respirations. Hyperventilation is a common occurrence in the dental office, as it is almost always the result of an episode of anxiety or emotional stress. Therefore, the prevention of hypertension is achieved by recognition and management of patient anxiety. Patients who admit to anxiety do not usually experience hyperventilation. A patient who is helped to deal with fear will not succumb to episodes of hyperventilation.

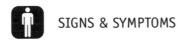 SIGNS & SYMPTOMS

Dizziness

Light-headedness

Numb fingers

Heart dysrhythmias

Abdominal cramps

Muscle cramps

Hyperventilation

 TREATMENT

Terminate dental treatment

Reassure the patient

Try to institute regular respirations

Rebreath exhalations to reverse alkalosis

Hypoglycemia

 INTRO

Hypoglycemia is a condition of acutely decreased blood sugar. A life-threatening condition, hypoglycemia is more critical than hyperglycemia in an emergency situation. Administration of glucose is indicated even if a definitive diagnosis is not made. Hypoglycemia must be treated rapidly. On the other hand, administration of glucose in a hyperglycemic crisis will not significantly affect the patient.

Hypoglycemia

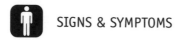 SIGNS & SYMPTOMS

Hunger

Nausea

Cool, moist skin

Shallow respirations

Irritation

Confusion

Bizarre behavior

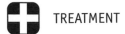 **TREATMENT**

Terminate procedure

Administer glucose

    Oral—paste or drink

    IV—5% D5W

Perform basic life support

Transport to hospital

Intraoral Lacerations

 INTRO

Although fortunately rare, intraoral lacerations do occur when treating patients. While efficient at cutting tooth structure, high-speed handpieces can also be efficient at cutting the soft tissue of the mouth. Because of the rich vascularity of the head and neck, intraoral lacerations can bleed extensively.

SIGNS & SYMPTOMS

Bleeding

    Pulsation, bright red—arterial

    Oozing, dark red—venous

Pain at trauma site or over area of swelling

Swelling—slowly or rapidly enlarging

Ecchymosis

Intraoral Lacerations

 TREATMENT

The procedure should be discontinued

Any foreign bodies should be removed from the mouth

Pressure should be applied to the trauma site with sterile gauze

Any foreign bodies should be removed from the wound

The wound should be flushed and irrigated with normal saline

Most bleeding from intraoral lacerations can be controlled with gauze pressure and isolated interrupted sutures

The addition of a hemostatic agent, such as absorbable gelatin sponges or oxidized cellulose with gauze under pressure, can be a valuable tool in controlling bleeding

Any bleeding vessels should be isolated, cross-clamped, and tied off with a suture

Bony bleeding can be controlled with application of gauze under pressure and, if needed, a hemostatic agent

Use of local anesthetic with a vasoconstrictor to control active bleeding should be discouraged because of the possibility of rebound bleeding after the vasoconstrictor wears off

INTRO

Myocardial infarction occurs when myocardial oxygen demand exceeds available oxygen supplied by the blood for an extended period. Patients suffering from coronary artery disease or atherosclerosis have plaques in their coronary arteries. These plaques can grow large enough to occlude the vessel, thereby decreasing blood flow to the oxygen-starved myocardium and causing myocardial ischemia. When the ischemia is prolonged, the myocardium is irreversibly damaged over the distribution of the occluded vessel. Most myocardial infarctions are a result of atherosclerotic coronary artery disease; however, vasospastic or Prinzmetal angina can cause decreased coronary artery blood flow.

Myocardial Infarction

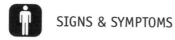 SIGNS & SYMPTOMS

Chest pain

    Crushing

    Radiating to neck, jaw, arm, back

    Substernal

Hypertension or hypotension

Indigestion

Diaphoresis (sweating)

Shortness of breath

Tachycardia or bradycardia

Dysrhythmias

Loss of or alteration in consciousness

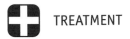 TREATMENT

Discontinue dental treatment

Place patient in a semireclined position

Administer supplemental oxygen

Continually monitor and record vital signs

Administer sublingual nitroglycerin, 0.4 mg every 5 minutes for three doses

Assume that the patient is having an infarction if he or she continues to have symptoms after the administration of three doses of nitroglycerin

Notify rescue unit and prepare for transport

Transport patient to the hospital as soon as possible

ADVANCED TREATMENT

Start IV with normal saline solution

Monitor ECG and treat dysrhythmias according to advanced cardiac life support protocols

Administer morphine, 1 to 6 mg IV, to relieve pain and anxiety and to decrease systemic vascular afterload

Myocardial Infarction

ACUTE MYOCARDIAL INFARCTION

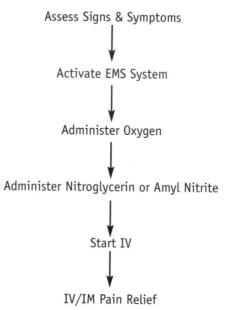

Assess Signs & Symptoms

↓

Activate EMS System

↓

Administer Oxygen

↓

Administer Nitroglycerin or Amyl Nitrite

↓

Start IV

↓

IV/IM Pain Relief

INTRO

Although rare, ocular injuries in the dental office do occur and require the same prompt attention as other more commonplace dental emergencies. Most ocular injuries occurring in the dental office are as a result of trauma to the cornea or the globe itself. Although not life-threatening, these injuries require rapid attention to minimize loss of visual acuity. Often, after initial treatment of these injuries, patients should be referred to an ophthalmologist for definitive treatment.

Ocular Injuries

Chemical Burns

Although any chemical burn can be serious, alkali burns are true emergencies.

 SIGNS & SYMPTOMS

Mild to severe pain

Blurred vision

Excessive tearing

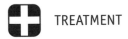 TREATMENT

Immediate copious irrigation with tap water

Alkali burns in particular require 15 to 20 minutes of copious irrigation before the patient is transported to a qualified physician

Copious irrigation before transportation is also indicated in acid burns

Prompt consultation and evaluation by an ophthalmologist

Ocular Injuries

Corneal Abrasions

Corneal abrasions are the most common ocular injury sustained in the dental office.

 SIGNS & SYMPTOMS

Mild to severe pain

Excessive tearing

Blurred vision

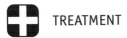 TREATMENT

Place double patch over affected eye

Refer to ophthalmologist for comprehensive slit-lamp evaluation with fluorescein dye

Administer topical antibiotics and analgesics after confirming diagnosis

Ocular Injuries

Foreign Bodies

 SIGNS & SYMPTOMS

Mild to moderate pain

Excessive tearing

Blurred vision as a result of tearing

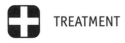 TREATMENT

Unless easily accessible, foreign bodies within the eye should be removed by a trained physician

The eye should be irrigated for nonembedded foreign material

If removal is decided against, the eye should be patched and the patient sent for slit-lamp examination by an ophthalmologist

Seizures

 INTRO

A seizure is a sudden and unexpected central paroxysmal neuronal depolarization of nerve cells that can result in uncontrolled muscular movement. Seizures take on two different forms: focal and generalized. Focal seizures are more limited in their progression or spread, usually without significant loss of consciousness. Generalized seizures have a more poorly defined origin and commonly result in a loss of consciousness. Generalized or grand mal seizures can be dramatic in presentation, whereas focal or partial seizures are less conspicuous. Seizures can be caused by many things, such as head injuries, high fevers, infections, neoplasms, cerebrovascular disease, and systemic conditions, or they can be idiopathic. Status epilepticus is a prolonged seizure, usually lasting more than 5 to 10 minutes, and fortunately is rare.

SIGNS & SYMPTOMS

Feeling of an aura-visual, auditory, or olfactory sensory disturbance

Minor personality changes

Depression

Anxiety

Headache

Memory loss

Loss of consciousness

Hallucinations

Uncontrolled muscle motor movements (tonic/colonic movements)

Extremity muscle rigidity

Shortness of breath

Tachycardia

Nystagmus

Urinary incontinence

Postictal (recovery) phase

Slow return of consciousness

Slow recovery

Sleepiness

Confusion

Disorientation

Amnesia

Seizures

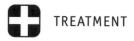 TREATMENT

Place patient in a reclined or supine position

Protect patient from injury during uncontrolled movements

Protect head from injury during seizure movements

Administer supplemental oxygen

Suction mouth secretions

Turn head to side if vomiting occurs and clear airway

Monitor vital signs

Initiate basic cardiac life support if indicated

Transport patient to nearest hospital if indicated

Provide transportation home—do not let patients drive themselves home

In cases of status epilepticus, start IV and administer diazepam IV and titrate to seizure control to maximum of 10 to 15 mg.

INTRO

Shock is defined as a condition in which the circulatory system inadequately perfuses the body tissues, resulting in cellular hypoxia. Shock is classified into several different types.

Hypovolemic shock is due to a sudden and acute loss of blood usually secondary to trauma. As blood is lost, intravascular volume is diminished, thereby reducing perfusion pressure and decreasing blood flow to vital organs and tissues.

Septic shock is due to the vasodilatory action of endotoxins produced by a virulent systemic bacteremia. Vasodilatation increases intravascular volume and decreases perfusion pressures.

Cardiogenic shock is a failure of the heart to pump a sufficient volume of blood to maintain perfusion pressure. This can be caused by myocardial infarction, heart valve failure, and cardiomyopathy.

Neurogenic shock is most often a result of spinal cord trauma causing loss of sympathetic stimulation, which in turn causes vasodilatation.

Shock

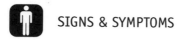 SIGNS & SYMPTOMS

Hypotension/postural hypotension

Tachycardia

Cool skin

Pale skin color

Anxiety

Change in mental status

Decrease capillary refill

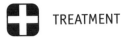 TREATMENT

The goal of treatment is to maintain perfusion pressure and thereby maintain oxygenation to vital organs and tissues.

Perform continual monitoring of vital signs

Monitor skin signs and capillary perfusion

Place patient in a supine position

Elevate the lower extremities

Provide supplemental oxygen

Transport patient to the closest hospital emergency room

Start large-bore IV

Replace fluid with normal saline or lactated Ringer's solution

Syncope

 INTRO

Vasodepressor syncope, commonly known as fainting, is a frequent occurrence during stressful situations, which include the delivery of dental care. This condition is usually benign; however, if left untreated, it can be fatal. The common faint is caused by a transitory and sudden loss of consciousness following a period of cerebral ischemia. Patients usually fall to the floor or are placed in a supine position, which results in restoration of blood flow and return to consciousness. If the flow patterns to the brain are not restored, however, life-threatening cardiovascular and pulmonary effects can occur.

Predisposing factors that can lead to syncope include fright, pain, emotional stress, anxiety, hunger, sudden postural changes, and exhaustion. Identifying these predisposing conditions and treating them can often prevent an episode of syncope.

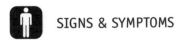 SIGNS & SYMPTOMS

Early

Loss of color, pallor

Perspiration

Nausea

Increased heart rate

Feeling of warmth

Late

Yawning

Dilated pupils

Cold extremities

Hypotension

Dizziness

Loss of consciousness

Syncope

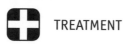 **TREATMENT**

Position patient—supine, head lower than feet if possible

Maintain open airway

Administer oxygen

Administer ammonia inhalant

Monitor vital signs

Legal Aspects to Emergency Medicine

Informed Consent, the Good Samaritan, and Malpractice

SCOTT D. BRAUN

The threat of a lawsuit is a significant concern overshadow-
ing a doctor's practice. Thus, it is essential for a doctor to
have some basic understanding of the law. This understanding will not only provide protection against a lawsuit, but
can also be a tool to assist in providing the patient with an
optimum level of care. It is often assumed that these two
goals are mutually exclusive. They are not. In fact, they are
complementary. Doctors and other health-care providers
need to understand that the technical requirements of the
law can be instrumental in providing the best possible care.
Too often, doctors regard the procedures mandated by the
law (and, as is more often the case, the doctor's attorney)
as a nuisance that interferes with patient care. A more dangerous concern is the belief that merely following rote procedure will provide absolute protection from a lawsuit. This
is not necessarily the case. Knowledge of the law and the
reasons why it mandates certain procedures can provide protection from a lawsuit but, more importantly, should be considered a tool to enhance patient care.

This chapter provides a general overview of some basic
principles underlying a malpractice lawsuit and takes a more
comprehensive look at two legal concepts that arise in emergency care situations: Good Samaritan Acts and the doctrine
of informed consent. The information contained in this chapter is meant to provide a general overview of common legal
principles and is not, nor should it be construed as, a com-

prehensive or authoritative statement of the law. It should be emphasized that although these concepts are generally accepted, the law of each particular jurisdiction provides the source of authority for any of the concepts discussed herein.

BASIC PRINCIPLES INVOLVED IN A MEDICAL MALPRACTICE SUIT

Generally, a medical malpractice suit is brought by a plaintiff (the patient) against a defendant (the doctor or other health-care professional) in a civil court, with the plaintiff seeking damages for an injury allegedly sustained in the course of medical treatment. The predominant theory of recovery in medical malpractice actions is negligence. In a negligence action, the plaintiff has the burden of proving each of the following elements by a preponderance of evidence:

1. The existence of a duty owed to the plaintiff by the doctor based on the doctor-patient relationship
2. A breach of the duty or standard of care
3. A compensable injury
4. A causal connection, consisting of the actual or cause-in-fact and proximate cause, between the injury and the act

A doctor's duty to his or her patient is embodied in the standard of care. The standard of care establishes the minimal level of care that the patient is entitled to while being treated by the doctor. Because a doctor possesses special skills, training, and knowledge, a special standard of care is used to determine whether a doctor acted negligently. The standard of care is usually stated as follows: a doctor must exercise the average degree of skill, care, and diligence exercised by members of the same profession.

Several issues arise in the context of a discussion of the standard of care. First, because it is assumed that the average person would not be capable of understanding the complex issues involved in most health-care issues, the standard of care is not defined by laypersons. Rather, expert testimony is required to define the standard of care in every malpractice lawsuit. Thus, the plaintiff is required to provide an expert to testify that the conduct of the defendant professional did not comply with generally accepted practice and procedure. Without such testimony, the plaintiff's case cannot proceed.

In an emergency situation, the plaintiff's burden is essentially the same. However, the law recognizes that in an emergency situation the treatment and care provided by a doctor may be quite different than that in a nonemergency situation. Thus, the plaintiff must establish that the doctor did not exercise the average degree of skill, care, and diligence exercised by members of the same profession in the same or similar emergency situation.

A related issue concerns the increased specialization in medical fields. It is generally recognized by the courts that the standard is that of the reasonable specialist. Thus, the applicable standard of care is increasingly that of the reasonable specialist (i.e., oral surgeon, orthodontist, endodontist). Also, the standard of care is no longer confined to the local geographic area within which the professional practices. It is thought that the proliferation and availability of the latest technology and information regarding care and treatment allow for the application of a national standard.

GOOD SAMARITAN STATUTES

Good Samaritan, or hold-harmless statutes, commonly arise in discussions of liability in emergency care situations. These statutes generally provide for immunity from civil prosecution to those rendering care in emergency situations. Generally, there is no duty to come to the aid of another. Thus, there is no requirement in the law to save a drowning person or bandage a bleeding person on the sidewalk. More importantly, the law imposes no special duty on doctors or other health-care professionals to come to the aid of others.

Similarly, physicians and other doctors are not required to enter into a doctor-patient relationship to provide their services or expertise to anyone at anytime. Generally, health-care professionals possess the right to refuse treatment to anyone for any reason, even in emergency situations. The touchstone of a medical malpractice action is the doctor-patient relationship. This special relationship gives rise to the duty of care owed by the doctor to the patient. As a result, there is a reluctance on the part of doctors to voluntarily provide care if by doing so they would create a special relationship giving rise to the potential for liability.

The purpose of the Good Samaritan statutes is to encourage health-care providers to render care voluntarily, by immunizing them from tort actions for negligent harm they cause to the victim/patient. The rationale behind such statutes is to promote social welfare by eliminating the threat of lawsuits.

These statutes vary in their scope from state to state. However, a common feature of these acts is that the services must be provided free of charge. Additionally, gross negligence, or willful or wanton misconduct, is not covered under most immunity statutes. *Black's Law Dictionary* defines gross negligence as: "The intentional failure to perform a manifest duty in reckless disregard of the consequences as affecting the life of another. A conscious voluntary act or omission likely to result in grave injury."

The definition of emergency, including what one consists of and where one occurs, also varies depending on each particular statute. Generally, these statutes provide for immunity "at the scene of" an emergency. Where is the scene of an emergency? Does this include an office setting or hospital? The answer depends on where one practices. Several courts have examined this issue and have come to different conclusions. Obviously, emergencies encountered outside a hospital on the street would be covered. Some courts that have considered the issue have held that physicians not on call, and having no prior relationship with the patient, responding to emergencies inside a hospital are covered by the statute. However, most courts define the scene of an emergency as excluding hospitals, offices, and other health-care facilities.

Generally, the question of whether an emergency situation existed is a question of fact decided by the trier of fact (either the judge or the jury). Thus, there is no standard answer. However, emergency situations have been construed very broadly, including situations occurring after a crisis has been stabilized. Additionally, the subjective belief of the health-care professional who provided the treatment can be taken into consideration. Clearly, an "emergency" caused by the actions of a provider during the course of treatment is not covered under these acts. However, they may provide a defense if the emergency care is provided to someone other than the patient. For example, treating a patient's relative in the waiting room of an office is probably covered.

INFORMED CONSENT

The legal doctrine of informed consent is a well-known legal issue in the health-care arena. Informed consent is a person's agreement to allow a medical intervention that is based on full disclosure of the facts needed to make the decision. Its purpose is to allow the patient to make an intelligent, or informed, decision about a specific course of treatment. Presumably, it is the patient's right to balance the risks and benefits of a particular intervention and make a decision whether to proceed. The aim of the doctrine of informed consent is to promote the patient's best interest and prevent the doctor from overreaching. This idea was first articulated in *Schloendorff v. Society of New York Hospital,* 211 N.Y. 125, 105 N.E. 92 (1914), which set forth the proposition that every adult person has a right of individual self-determination regarding health care.

The roots of the doctrine of informed consent lie in the common law tort of battery. In common law, battery is an intentional act consisting of the nonconsensual harmful or offensive touching of another person. There is no requirement that the contact cause physical damage. Thus, in a treatment situation, any action that is taken without the patient's consent, or that exceeds the scope of the consent originally given, is technically battery. However, the legal theory behind the doctrine has been broadened to include negligence. In these situations, the patient claims that the health-care provider is guilty of negligent nondisclosure of information.

Accordingly, there are two distinct types of informed consent claims. First, a patient may have a cause of action against the doctor for failing to obtain consent. This cause of action is viable even if the provider has performed the treatment properly within the standard of medical care. In these situations, the cause of action arises against the provider for failing to obtain the patient's knowledgeable consent to the treatment or providing treatment after consent is withdrawn. In *Bailey v. Belinfante*, 135 Ga. App.574, 218 S.E. 2d 289 (Court of Georgia Appeals 1975), a plaintiff brought a cause of action for battery against an oral surgeon who extracted 27 of the plaintiff's teeth. In this case, the patient had given valid consent regarding the extraction of only 11 teeth. Thus, the removal of the extra 16 teeth, although medically necessary and performed competently, constituted technical battery.

The second and most prevalent type of informed consent claim involves the lack of disclosure of adequate information. This type of claim involves a negligence action when consent is given but is not supported by adequate disclosure of information to the patient.

There are two competing standards to determine whether consent is informed enough to be legally effective. The first is a more traditional, physician-based standard. Under this standard, the doctor's duty of disclosure is measured by reference to other professionals, like a traditional malpractice standard. It is the duty of the doctor to disclose what a reasonable doctor would disclose under the same or similar circumstances. This standard presumes that adequate disclosure is a medical judgment best made by a medical professional.

A more modern standard shifts the focus to the patient. Under this approach, the duty of disclosure is defined by what the patient would want to know, rather than what the provider thinks the patient should know. Under this approach, consent is valid only if the provider discloses all material risks of treatment, alternative treatments, or the consequences of no treatment at all. This standard mandates that the choice to undergo treatment be the patient's, not the provider's. A plurality of states have adopted the patient-based approach, whereas a lesser minority has retained the physician-based standard.

Who Can Give Valid Consent?

Obviously, the duty of disclosure is owed to the patient. In most situations, the patient undergoing the proposed treatment is the only person qualified to give consent. In some situations, this is not the case. One of the most frequent questions asked by practitioners is, "Who is capable of giving the required consent to treatment?"

It is a presumption in the law that, absent evidence to the contrary, a patient is in possession of sufficient faculties and mental capabilities to understand the information being given and can exercise independent judgment as to whether he or she will undergo the proposed procedure. Thus, in most cases, the patient can give consent, and the health-care provider must abide by the decision of the patient.

However, there are special rules for patients who are deemed incompetent to give valid consent. In these situations, competence is not presumed. First, patients who have been adjudicated as incompetent by a court of competent jurisdiction are unable to give valid consent. The substantive and procedural requirements of such a proceeding vary from state to state. In this situation, valid consent can only be given by the patient's legal guardian or by an order of a court.

A second category of patients the law deems legally incompetent to give consent are minors. In common law, the age of majority was 21 years. However, most states have passed statutes lowering the age of majority to 18 years. Of course, there are exceptions to this general proposition. A "mature minor," or legally emancipated minor, is a person who has not attained the legal age of majority but has sufficient discretion and intellectual capacity to give legally effective consent. Minors who are married, in the armed services, or females with children are examples of mature minors.

The most difficult situation for a health-care provider to assess is when the patient is of questionable competence. In these situations, if it is not obvious that the patient falls into one of the above categories of incompetents, then the health-care provider is placed in the difficult position of judging whether the patient can give adequate consent, or refusal, to undergo the proposed medical intervention. It is important to remember that the law presumes that a person is competent. In these situations, the best protection, although not the most practical, is an order from a court. However, in most cases, this option is not feasible. The next best option is to consult with other medical professionals. Most large health-care facilities provide for procedures for administrative consent. Lastly, it is good practice to involve the patient's relatives in the decision-making process if possible.

Another large area of concern and confusion arises when the patient is unable to give valid consent. As noted above, both the Constitution and common law recognize a right of privacy and individual self-determination regarding a person's health. This right is derived from the patient, not others. However, the law has recognized several situations in which persons other than the patient can give valid consent to treatment.

For example, the law has recognized the validity of emergency consent in situations in which prompt medical attention is required because of delirium, unconsciousness, or other disability. In these situations, valid consent to medical procedures can be obtained from the patient's next-of-kin, a legal representative, or a health-care provider. A health-care provider who encounters a patient who is in serious distress and unable to consent is entitled to presume, absent evidence to the contrary, that the patient would wish to receive medically appropriate treatment, at least to the extent necessary to preserve life or prevent serious consequences of nontreatment.

The scope of the emergency consent differs from jurisdiction to jurisdiction. For example, some states' statutes allow medical intervention only when the patient is confronted with a life-threatening emergency. Some allow intervention to relieve pain and suffering, whereas others allow intervention only when the threat to the patient is immediate and only to the extent truly necessary to preserve life.

Generally, a requirement for valid emergency consent is the existence of a bona fide emergency. The definition of emergency varies from state to state. Also, the health-care professional must make attempts to reach the patient's next-of-kin to obtain proxy consent. Lastly, the care rendered must be consistent with recognized professional standards and limited to that necessary to deal with the emergency at hand.

Next-of-kin or proxy consent is a central concept in the analysis of emergency consent. It is generally accepted that in emergency situations, decision-making power regarding treatment passes to the patient's next-of-kin. Of course, the feasibility of contacting a patient's next-of-kin will always depend on the nature of the emergency situation. It is important to ascertain who is the patient's closest relative. It is that person who has the power to give the necessary consent. If proxy consent is obtained over the telephone, it may be advisable to tape-record the authorization or have the person repeat the authorization to another health-care provider.

What Makes Consent Informed?

Several information items must be disclosed to the patient before a proposed procedure is undertaken, including diagnosis and prognosis, nature and purpose, risks and consequences, and alternative treatments. First and perhaps most obvious, a diagnosis of the patient's condition should always be communicated to the patient. Second, a description of the nature and purpose of the proposed treatment should be provided. This need not, however, include the specific details of how the procedure is going to be performed. Third, a health-care provider needs to provide an assessment of the risks and consequences of a proposed procedure. Although it is too time-consuming to disclose all possible risks, adequate disclosure is a function of the probability that a risk will actually occur as well as the severity of the risk. Those risks that have a high probability of occurrence and remote risks that have severe consequences should always be disclosed. Risks that are very remote or commonly known need not be disclosed.

Providing a patient with information about alternative treatments, including delaying or forgoing the proposed medical intervention, is a very important aspect of providing adequate information. All reasonably feasible alternatives to treatment should be disclosed even if they are beyond the capabilities of the primary health-care provider. A health-care provider must give the patient enough information about alternative opportunities so that he or she can explore them. However, an in-depth discourse on alternative treatments is not necessary. The patient need only be made aware that different options to treatment exist.

Lastly, there are several other information items that, although not technically required, help to adequately inform the patient. These include the cost, length of recovery, and level of pain involved in the proposed procedure. Also, insurance coverage information is often an area of patient concern. Further, some jurisdictions have required that the caregiver provide his or her qualifications to perform the proposed treatment. This can include whether the caregiver suffers from alcoholism or is HIV positive.

What Happens if the Procedure Varies From What Was Described?

At times a doctor may discover an unexpected situation or condition that requires procedures to be expanded beyond the scope originally contemplated and agreed to by the patient. In these surprise situations, the extension doctrine allows for the extension of a procedure to include aspects not originally contemplated. In these situations, the doctor will not be liable for the performance of an unauthorized operation. Obviously, it is impractical to interrupt a procedure to obtain additional consent. Also, this doctrine allows the provider, who is already familiar with the patient's condition, a measure of latitude to achieve the goals of the medical intervention.

There are some limitations to the scope of the extension doctrine. It does not apply to situations in which the possible need to expand or extend the procedure should have been originally contemplated by the patient's doctor. Additionally, there must be an urgent need to expand the procedure, necessitated by the surprise nature of the newly found condition. The extension doctrine does not provide protection in situations in which it would be possible to obtain the patient's consent to the expanded procedure. Generally, courts do not look with favor on blanket authorizations. Thus, as a practical matter, consent forms should not be worded in terms of correcting broad conditions, but rather in terms of specific procedures.

Are There Situations When Full Disclosure Is Not Required?

Although the doctrine of informed consent rests on the idea of full disclosure to the patient, there are times when full disclosure may not be required. For instance, patients are free to decide not to receive information about their condition or treatment. The law does not require a provider to force disclosure of information on patients. However, the decision not to receive any information must be made freely and be supported by adequate knowledge. Also, the waiver must be a voluntary, informed choice—basically, informed consent in reverse.

As noted above, very remote risks and well-known risks need not be disclosed. However, an individual patient's condition and characteristics must be considered when making this determination. This includes not only the patient's medical condition, but also background, education, and professional level. Thus, the quantity and substance of information given to a layperson may differ dramatically from that given to another health-care professional.

Perhaps the most well-known principle providing for less than full disclosure is the therapeutic privilege. The law recognizes that at times it may be appropriate for doctors to withhold information when, from a medical standpoint, it is in the patient's best interest. This privilege is based on the assumption that, with full knowledge of the situation, a negative outcome might occur. Of course, the decision to withhold information based on the therapeutic privilege should be accurately documented.

Finally, there are several practical issues concerning informed consent that will be helpful to examine. Proper documentation is a significant tool in proving that the provider has met all required legal obligations. It is important to develop thorough and consistent procedures for documenting consent. Good documentation procedures cannot only provide protection from a lawsuit, but can also enhance patient care. However, it cannot be emphasized enough that documentation is not a panacea. The presence of a signed form is not a magic shield that automatically provides protection from a lawsuit. In most jurisdictions, there is no legal requirement that consent must be written to be valid. On the bright side, the absence of a written form does not sound the death knell for the provider. Further, whereas proper documentation can be very helpful, improper or incomplete forms can be dangerous. If the form does not expressly mention an item of information that was in fact conveyed to the patient but was not recorded, the patient has a much easier time claiming that it was omitted.

Another issue that often arises in urban practice settings is language. Often, a provider must treat a patient who has little or no understanding of English. Generally, a provider should take all reasonable feasible measures to provide the patient with as much information as possible. This may include translation through a family member or other office worker. As always, it is important to document what steps were taken to provide the patient with information.

Finally, there is no fixed time limit once valid consent has been given. It is obvious that the more time that passes between the initial consent and subsequent interventions, the more its validity becomes suspect. The patient's condition may change dramatically between the initial consent and the intervention. Material changes in a patient's condition erode the knowing and voluntary requirements of an initial informed consent. Thus, it is the better practice to obtain consent before each intervention.

SECTION IV.

Tables

Abbreviations Used in Prescription Writing

a—before	ac—before	ad lib—as desired, as
bid—twice a day	food (meals)	much as
		wanted
d—day	c̄—with	cap—capsule
gtt—drop	disp—dispense	gm—gram
hs—at bedtime	gr—grain	h—hour
po—by mouth	no—number	p̄—after
qh—every hour	prn—as required,	pc—after food
q4h—every 4 hours	if needed	qd—every day
tab—tablet	qid—4 times a day	sig—write (label)
	s̄—without	stat—immediately
	tid—3 times a day	(now)

Approximate Equivalents (Metric and Apothecaries)

1 mg = 1/60 gr			500 mL = 1 pt
30 gm = 1 oz	30 mg = 0.5 gr	1 kg = 2.2 lb	1000 mL = 1 qt
1 gm = 15 gr	60 mg = 1 gr	1 kg = 1000 gm	454 gm = 1 lb

Common Household Equivalents

1 drop (gtt)—0.05 mL	1 teaspoon (tsp)—5 mL	1 tablespoon (tbsp)—15 mL

Sample Prescription Form

John Doe, D.D.S.   (123) 456-7890
123 Molar Way, #1
Anywhere, USA 54321-1234

DATE _____

NAME _____AGE _____

ADDRESS_____

℞ *Name of drug and size of tablet or capsule or concentration of liquid*

DISP: *The number of tablets or capsules or quantity of liquid to be dispensed (number of refills should be noted)*

SIG: *Instruction on how to take or use the medication*

_____D.D.S.	_____D.D.S.
Dispense as written	Product selection permitted

DEA # *Required for class II, III, IV, V drugs* (should not be preprinted on prescription pad)

Analgesics Used in Dentistry

			Brand Name	Generic Name
Over the counter			Bayer 325 mg	Acetylsalicylic acid (ASA)
			Anacin	ASA 400 mg Caffeine 32 mg
			Tylenol 325 mg, 500 mg	Acetaminophen
			Motrin 200 mg	Ibuprofen
			Aleve 220 mg	Naproxen sodium
Federal Law Prohibits Dispensing Without a Prescription	No DEA number required	Nonscheduled	Dolobid 250 mg, 500 mg	Diflunisal
			Motrin 400 mg, 600 mg, 800 mg	Ibuprofen
			Ansaid 50 mg, 100 mg	Flubiprofen
			Ultram 50 mg	Tramadol hydrochloride
			Toradol 10 mg	Ketorolac tromethamine
	DEA number required, up to 5 refills, can be telephoned to pharmacy	IV	Darvocet-N-100	Proproxyphene napsylate 100 mg Acetaminophen 650 mg
			Talwin NX 50 mg	Pentazocine hydrochloride 50 mg Naloxone hydrochloride 0.5 mg
		CLASS III	Tylenol #2, #3, #4	Codeine phosphate 15, 30, 60 mg Acetaminophen 300 mg
			Empirin #2, #3, #4	Codeine phosphate 15, 30, 60 mg ASA 325 mg
			DHCplus	Dihydrocodeine bitarate 16 mg Caffeine 30 mg Acetaminophen 356 mg
			Vicodin	Hydrocodone bitarate 5 mg Acetaminophen 500 mg
			Vicodin ES	Hydrocodone bitarate 7.5 mg Acetaminophen 750 mg
			Lortab 2.5,10	Hydrocodone bitarate 2.5, 5.0 mg Acetaminophen 500 mg
			Lortab 7.5,	Hydrocodone bitarate 7.5, 10 mg Acetaminophen 500 mg
			Lorcet HD	Hydrocodone bitarate 5.0 mg Acetaminophen 500 mg
			Lorcet PLUS 10/650	Hydrocodone bitarate 7.5, 10 mg Acetaminophen 650 mg
	DEA number and triplicate form required	CLASS II	Percodan	Oxycodone hydrochloride 4.5 mg Oxycodone terephthlate 0.38 mg ASA 325 mg
			Percodan-demi	Oxycodone hydrochloride 2.25 mg Oxycodone terephthlate 0.19 mg ASA 325 mg
			Percocet	Oxycodone hydrochloride 5 mg Acetaminophen 325 mg
			Tylox	Oxycodone hydrochloride 5 mg Acetaminophen 500 mg
			Dilaudid 1 mg, 2 mg, 3 mg, 4 mg	Hydromorphone hydrochloride

Instructions	Maximum Daily Dose
1–2 tabs q4h	4000 mg
1–2 tabs q4–6h	4000 mg
1–2 tabs q4–6h	4000 mg
1–4 tabs q6–8h	3200 mg
2 tabs then 1 tab q8–12h	1375 mg
2 tabs then 1 tab q8–12h	1500 mg
up to 800 mg q6h	3200 mg
50–100 mg q6–8h	300 mg
50–100 mg q4–6h	400 mg
1 tab q4–6h	4 tabs
1 tab q4h	6 tabs
1 tab q3–4h	12 tabs
1–2 tabs q4h	360 mg 4000 mg
1–2 tabs q4h	360 mg 4000 mg
1–2 tabs q4h	12 caps
1–2 tabs q4–6h	8 tabs
1 tab q6h	6 tabs
1–2 tabs q4–6h	8 tabs
1 tab q6h	6 tabs
1–2 tabs q4–6h	8 tabs
1 tab q6h	6 tabs
1 tab q6h	6 tabs
1–2 tabs q6h	12 tabs
1 tab q6h	6 tabs
1 cap q6h	4 caps
2 mg q4–6h	24 mg

Anesthetic Milligram Conversion Table

Concentration		Cartridges (1.8 cc)											
% or Ratio	mg/cc	1	2	3	4	5	6	7	8	9	10	11	12
Anesthetic component													
0.5	5 mg	9	18	27	36	45	54	63	72	81	90	99	108
1.5%	15 mg	27	54	81	108	135	162	189	216	252	270	297	324
2%	20 mg	36	72	108	144	180	216	252	288	324	360	396	432
3%	30 mg	54	108	162	216	270	324	378	432	486	540	594	648
4%	40 mg	72	144	216	288	360	432	504	576	648	720	792	868
Vasoconstrictor (epinephrine, levonordefrin, levoarterenol)													
1:20,000	0.05 mg	0.09	0.18	0.27	0.36	0.45	0.54	0.63	0.72	0.81	0.90	0.99	0.108
1:30,000	0.033 mg	0.059	0.118	0.178	0.237	0.245	0.354	0.413	0.475	0.531	0.590	0.649	0.708
1:50,000	0.02 mg	0.036	0.072	0.108	0.144	0.180	0.216	0.252	0.288	0.324	0.360	0.396	0.432
1:100,000	0.01 mg	0.018	0.036	0.054	0.072	0.09	0.108	0.126	0.144	0.162	0.180	0.198	0.216
1:200,000	0.005 mg	0.009	0.018	0.027	0.036	0.045	0.054	0.063	0.072	0.081	0.09	0.099	0.108

Commonly Used Dental Anesthetics

Anesthetic				Vasoconstrictor						
Brand Name	Generic Manufacturer		Percentage-Concentration	Plain	1:50,000 Epinephrine	1:100,000 Epinephrine	1:200,000 Epinephrine	1:20,000 Levonordefrin	1:20,000 Neo-cobifrin	1:30,000 Levophed
Lidocaine										
Lidocaine HCL	Many generics		2%	X	X	X				
Alphacaine HCL	Carlisle Labs		2%		X	X				
Octocaine HCL	Novocol Chemical		2%	X	X	X				
Xylocaine HCL	Astra Pharmaceutical		2%	X	X	X				
Mepivacaine										
Mepivacaine HCL	Many generics		3%	X				X		2%
Arestocaine HCL	Carlisle Labs		3%	X				X		2%
Carbocaine HCL	Cook-Waite Labs		3%	X			X		X	2%
Isocaine HCL	Novocol Chemical		3%	X				X		2%
Polocaine HCL	Astra Pharmaceutical		3%	X				X		2%
Prilocaine										
Citanest Plain	Astra Pharmaceutical		4%	X						
Citanest Forte	Astra Pharmaceutical		4%				X			
Bupivacaine										
Marcaine HCL	Cook-Waite Labs		0.5%				X			
Etidocaine										
Duranest	Astra Pharmaceutical		1.5%				X			

continued

125

Commonly Used Dental Anesthetics

| Anesthetic | | | | | Vasoconstrictor | | | | | |
| Generic | Manufacturer | | | | 1: 50,000 Epine- phrine | 1: 100,000 Epine- phrine | 1: 200,000 Epine- phrine | 1: 20,000 Levonor- defrin | 1: 20,000 Neo- cobifrin | 1: 30,000 Levo- phed |
Brand Name		Percentage Concen- tration	Plain							
Propoxycaine[a]										
Ravocaine	Cook-Waite Labs						X			
Ravocaine	Cook-Waite Labs									X

Topical Anesthetic

Generic	Proprietary	Manufacturer
Benzocaine/tetracaine	Cetacaine 14%/2%	Cetylite Industries
	Gingicaine	Belport Co. Inc.
Butacaine sulfate	Butyn dental ointment 4%	Abbott Laboratories
Dyclonine HCL	Dyclone solution 0.5%	Merrell Dow Laboratories Inc.
Lidocaine HCL	Lidocaine gel 5%	Astra Pharmaceutical and Premier Dental Labs
	Lidocaine liquid 5%	Astra Pharmaceutical and Graham Chemical Corp.
	Lidocaine ointment 5%	Astra Pharmaceutical and Graham Chemical Corp.
	Lidocaine aerosol 10%	Astra Pharmaceutical
	Alphacaine ointment 5%	Carlisle Labs
	Octocaine ointment 5%	Novocol Chemical

Note: Topical anesthetic agents are absorbed systematically and must be considered when calculating the total anesthetic dosage.

[a]Available only in combination, 0.4% propoxycaine and 2% procaine.

Adult Dental Anesthetic Dosages

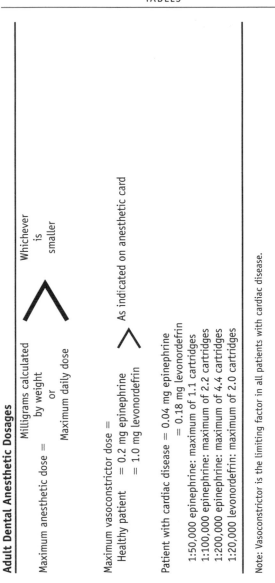

Maximum anesthetic dose =
Milligrams calculated by weight
or
Maximum daily dose
} Whichever is smaller

Maximum vasoconstrictor dose =
Healthy patient = 0.2 mg epinephrine
= 1.0 mg levonordefrin
} As indicated on anesthetic card

Patient with cardiac disease = 0.04 mg epinephrine
= 0.18 mg levonordefrin

1:50,000 epinephrine: maximum of 1.1 cartridges
1:100,000 epinephrine: maximum of 2.2 cartridges
1:200,000 epinephrine: maximum of 4.4 cartridges
1:20,000 levonordefrin: maximum of 2.0 cartridges

Note: Vasoconstrictor is the limiting factor in all patients with cardiac disease.

127

Pediatric Dental Anesthetic Dosages

Clark's rule

$$\text{Maximum dose for children} = \frac{\text{Child's weight (lb)}}{150} \times \text{Maximum recommended dose for adults}$$

Young's rule

$$\text{Child's dose} = \frac{\text{Adult dose}}{\text{Child's age} + 12/\text{Child's age}}$$

Adult Local Anesthetic Dosages[a]

Anesthetic agent	Patient weight in pounds (2.2 lb/kg)										
	50	60	70	80	90	100	110	120	130	140	150
2% Lidocaine (4.5 mg/kg, 2 mg/lb) Max dose 300 mg	100/2.7	120/3.3	140/3.8	160/4.4	180/5.0	200/5.5	220/6.1	240/6.6	260/7.2	280/7.7	300[b]/8.3
2% Lidocaine 1:100,000 epinephrine (7 mg/kg, 3.2 mg/lb) Max dose 500 mg	160/4.4	192/5.3	224/6.2	256/7.1	288/8.0	320/8.8	352/9.7	384/10.6	416/11.1[c]		
2% Lidocaine 1:50,000 epinephrine (7 mg/kg, 3.2 mg/lb) Max dose 500 mg	Recommended for hemostasis only. Maximum dose 5.5[c] cartridges for adults 100 lb or more										
3% Mepivacaine (4.4 mg/kg, 2 mg/lb) Max dose 300 mg	100/1.8	120/2.2	140/2.5	160/2.9	180/3.3	200/3.7	220/4.0	240/4.4	260/4.8	280/5.1	300[b]/5.5
2% Mepivacaine 1:20,000 levonordefrin (4.4 mg/kg, 2 mg/lb)	100/2.7	120/3.3	140/3.8	160/4.4	180/5.0	200/5.5	220/6.1	240/6.6	260/7.2	280/7.7	300[b]/8.3

continued

Adult Local Anesthetic Dosages[a]

	Patient weight in pounds (2.2 lb/kg)										
Anesthetic agent	50	60	70	80	90	100	110	120	130	140	150
1.5 Etidocaine 1:200,000 epinephrine (8 mg/kg, 3.6 mg/lb) Max dose 300 mg	180/6.6	216/8.0	252/9.3	288/10.6	324/12.0	360/13.3	396[b]/14.6				
4% Prilocaine with or without epinephrine (6 mg/kg, 2.7 mg/lb) Max dose 400 mg	135/1.8	162/2.2	189/2.6	216/3.0	243/3.3	270/3.7	297/4.1	324/4.5	351/4.8	378[b]/5.2	
0.5% Bupivacaine 1:200,000 epinephrine (1.3 mg/kg, 0.6 mg/lb) Max dose 90 mg	30/3.3	36/4.0	42/4.6	48/5.3	54/6.0	60/6.6	66/7.3	72/8.0	78/8.6	84/9.3	90[b]/10.0

[a]First number indicates number of milligrams. Second number indicates maximum cartridges (1.8 cc).

[b]Maximum dose regardless of weight.

[c]Vasoconstrictor limits dose.

Pediatric Local Anesthetic Dosages[7]

Anesthetic agent	Patient weight in pounds (2.2 lb/kg)										
	20	25	30	35	40	45	50	55	60	65	70
2% Lidocaine (4.5 mg/kg, 2 mg/lb) Max dose 300 mg	40/1.1	50/1.3	6C/1.6	70/1.9	80/2.2	90/2.5	100/2.7	110/3.0	120/3.3	130/3.6	140/3.8
2% Lidocaine 1:100,000 epinephrine (7 mg/kg, 3.2 mg/lb) Max dose 500 mg	64/1.7	80/2.2	96/2.6	112/3.1	128/3.5	144/4.0	160/4.4	176/4.8	192/5.3	208/5.7	224/6.2
2% Lidocaine 1:50,000 epinephrine (7 mg/kg, 3.2 mg/lb) Max dose 500 mg	Not recommended for children younger than 12										
3% Mepivacaine (4.4 mg/kg, 2 mg/lb) Max dose 300 mg	40/0.7	50/0.9	60/1.1	70/1.2	80/1.4	90/1.6	100/1.8	110/2.0	120/2.2	130/2.4	140/2.5
2% Mepivacaine 1:20,000 levonordefrin	40/1.1	50/1.3	60/1.6	70/1.9	80/2.2	90/2.5	100/2.7	110/3.0	120/3.3	130/3.6	140/3.8

continued

131

Pediatric Local Anesthetic Dosages[a]

Anesthetic agent	Patient weight in pounds (2.2 lb/kg)										
	20	25	30	35	40	45	50	55	60	65	70
1.5% Etidocaine 1:200,000 epinephrine (8 mg/kg, 3.6 mg/lb) Max dose 400 mg	72/2.6	90/3.3	108/4.0	126/4.6	144/5.3	162/6.0	180/6.6	198/7.3	216/8.0	234/8.6	252/9.3
(4.4 mg/lb, 2 mg/lb) (Max dose 300 mg)											
4% Prilocaine with or without epinephrine (6 mg/kg, 2.7 mg/lb) Max dose 400 mg	54/0.7	67/0.9	81/1.1	94/1.3	108/1.5	121/1.6	135/1.8	148/2.0	162/2.2	175/2.4	189/2.6
0.5% Bupivacaine 1:200,000 epinephrine (1.3 mg/kg, 0.6 mg/lb) Max dose 90 mg	Not recommended for children younger than 12										

[a] First number indicates number of milligrams. Second number indicates maximum cartridges (1.8 cc).

Mandibular Injections[a]

Injection	Area Anesthetized	Injection Site	Administration Technique[b]	Quantity
Inferior alveolar	All teeth Anterior gingiva Labial mucosa Lip	Center of pterygomandibular triangle (slightly posterior) Pterygomandibular raphae External oblique ridge Attachment of temporalis	Inject parallel to occlusal plane Inject from opposite premolar area Inject at level of lingual, bone contacted *Near mandibular foramen, 12–18 mm deep*	1–2 cartridges
Lingual	Lingual gingiva Tongue	Same as inferior alveolar	Retract needle halfway from inferior alveolar injection site *Along path of lingual nerve, 4–8 mm*	0.25–0.50 cartridges
Long buccal	Mucosa of cheek Gingiva buccal to molars	1 cm above occlusal plane between external and internal oblique ridges	Tip of needle advanced just through mucosa *Along path of buccal nerve*	0.25–0.50 cartridges
Mental	Anterior labial gingiva Labial mucosa Lip	Mucobuccal fold below first premolar	Tip of needle advanced just through mucosa *Near mental foramen*	0.25–0.50 cartridges
Incisive	Anterior teeth	Mental foramen, generally positioned apical to premolar teeth	Tip of needle adjacent to mental foramen Adjacent to mental foramen *(many feel the tip of the*	0.25–0.50 cartridges

continued

133

Mandibular Injections[a]

Injection	Area Anesthetized	Injection Site	Administration Technique[b]	Quantity
			needle must actually be in the mental canel to achieve adequate anesthesia)	
Gow-gates	Teeth Buccal and lingual gingiva Tongue Labial mucosa and lip	Adjacent to mesial lingual cusp of max second molar	Direct needle cross arch toward intratragel notch (requires wide opening) Advance until contact with neck of condyle *Along path of mandibular nerve*	1 cartridge
Akanosi	Teeth Buccal and lingual gingiva Tongue Labial mucosa and lip	Lingual to ramus At level of maxillary tuberosity	Mouth remains closed or nearly closed Advance needle parallel to medial surface of ramus *Along path of mandibular nerve, 25 mm deep*	1 cartridge
Periodontal ligament (PDL)	Any single tooth (maxillary or mandibular)	Gingival sulcus	Direct needle along axis of tooth into PDL space *Anesthetic forced under pressure into PDL space*	Minimal

[a]Anesthetic deposit locations in italics.

[b]Always aspirate before injecting.

Maxillary Injections[a]

Injection	Area Anesthetized	Injection Site	Administration Technique[b]	Quantity
Posterior superior alveolar (PSA)	Third molar Second molar Distobuccal root of first molar Buccal periodontium and bone	Height of mucobuccal fold above second molar	Upward 45° to the occlusal plane Inward and backward 45–90° to the midsaggital plane *Near foramen of PSA nerve, 12–18 mm deep, above apex of third molar*	1 cartridge
Middle superior alveolar (MSA)	First and second premolar Mesiobuccal root or first molar Buccal periodontium and bone	Height of mucobuccal fold above second molar	Parallel to long axis of second premolar above the apex of the root *Advance needle along bone until tip is above the second premolar, 6–12 mm deep*	1 cartridge
Anterior superior alveolar (ASA)	Central incisor Lateral incisor Cuspid Facial periodontium and bone	Height of mucobuccal fold mesial to root of cuspid above the lateral incisor in the canine fossa	Angle needle from lateral toward the bone above the apex of the cuspid *Above apex of cuspid, 6–12 mm deep*	1 cartridge
Infraorbital	Same as ASA Soft tissue of lower eyelid	Similar to ASA higher in canine fossa close to the infraorbital foramen	Angle needle slightly more medially than ASA, advance toward infraorbital rim	1 cartridge

continued

135

Maxillary Injections[a]

Injection	Area Anesthetized	Injection Site	Administration Technique[b]	Quantity
	Cheek Lateral aspect of nose		(palpate infraorbital rim + foramen) *Near the infraorbital foramen*	
Second division block	All maxillary teeth, bone, and soft tissue on side of injection	Greater palatine foramen Or similar to PSA	Direct needle up greater palatine canal Direct needle superior and medial through pterygo-palatine fissure *Pterygopalatine fossa (aspiration very important)*	1–2 cartridges
Greater palatine	Bone and soft tissue, posterior palate to mesial of first premolar, gingiva to midline of palate	Soft tissue slightly anterior to greater palatine foramen	Advance syringe from opposite side of mouth at right angles to target area *At junction of vertical and horizontal planes of hard palate, 5–7 mm deep*	0.25–0.50 cartridges
Nasopalatine	Bone and soft tissue, cupsid to cupsid on anterior palate	Either side of incisive papilla	45–90° to tissue adjacent to incisive papilla (watch for blanching) *Through soft tissue nest to incisive papilla, 3–5 mm deep*	0.25–0.50 cartridges

continued

Maxillary Injections[a]

Injection	Area Anesthetized	Injection Site	Administration Technique[b]	Quantity
Soft tissue anesthesia (any area)	Soft tissue adjacent to injection site	Adjacent to area requiring anesthesia	Direct needle into edge of wound or adjacent to area to be anesthetized *Wound edge, under lesion to be excised or area to be incised*	Variable

[a]Anesthetic deposit locations in italics.

[b]Always aspirate before injecting.

Suggested Readings

American Heart Association. Guidelines for cardiopulmonary resuscitation. JAMA 1992;268:2171.

Andreoli TE, Bennett JC, Carpenter CC, et al. Cecil essentials of medicine. Philadelphia: WB Saunders, 1993.

Fishman MC, Hoffman AR, Klausner RD, et al. Medicine. Philadelphia: JB Lippincott, 1985.

Malamed SF. Medical emergencies in the dental office. St. Louis: CV Mosby, 1993.

National Institute on Drug Abuse. National household survey on drug abuse. Rockville, MD: Department of Health and Human Services, 1993.

Rakel RE. Conn's current therapy. Philadelphia: WB Saunders, 1992.

Rose LF, Kaye D. Internal medicine for dentistry. St. Louis: CV Mosby, 1990.

Schwartz GR. Principles and practice of emergency medicine. Baltimore: Williams & Wilkins, 1998.

Yagiela JA, Neidle EA, Dowd FJ. Pharmacology and therapeutics for dentistry. St. Louis: CV Mosby, 1998.